CONFIDENCE PERSONIFIED

BUILDING SELF-ESTEEM

LERBERN M LERSON

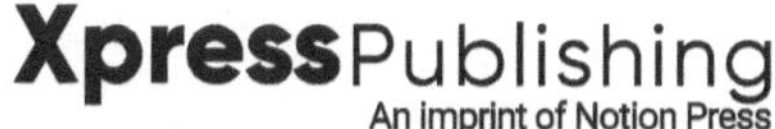

Xpress Publishing
An imprint of Notion Press

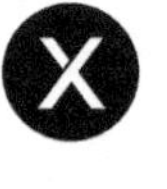

XpressPublishing
An imprint of Notion Press

No.8, 3rd Cross Street,CIT Colony,
Mylapore, Chennai, Tamil Nadu-600004

Copyright © Lerbern M Lerson
All Rights Reserved.

ISBN 978-1-63606-529-8

This book has been published with all efforts taken to make the material error-free after the consent of the author. However, the author and the publisher do not assume and hereby disclaim any liability to any party for any loss, damage, or disruption caused by errors or omissions, whether such errors or omissions result from negligence, accident, or any other cause.

While every effort has been made to avoid any mistake or omission, this publication is being sold on the condition and understanding that neither the author nor the publishers or printers would be liable in any manner to any person by reason of any mistake or omission in this publication or for any action taken or omitted to be taken or advice rendered or accepted on the basis of this work. For any defect in printing or binding the publishers will be liable only to replace the defective copy by another copy of this work then available.

Contents

Weight Loss

<u>**Here are many ways to lose a lot of weight fast.**</u>

- Many diet plans leave you feeling hungry or unsatisfied. These are major reasons why you might find it hard to stick to a diet.
- However, not all diets have this effect. Low carb diets are effective for weight loss and may be easier to stick to than other diets.
- Here's a 3-step weight loss plan that employs a low carb diet and aims to:
- significantly reduce your appetite
- cause fast weight loss
- improve your metabolic health at the same time

<u>1. Cut back on carbs</u>

- The most important part is to cut back on sugars and starches, or carbohydrates.
- When you do that, your hunger levels go down, and you generally end up eating significantly fewer calories (1).
- Instead of burning carbs for energy, your body now starts burning stored fat for energy.

- Another benefit of cutting carbs is that it lowers insulin levels, causing the kidneys to shed excess sodium and water. This reduces bloating and unnecessary water weight (2, 3Trusted Source).
- According to some dietitians, it's not uncommon to lose up to 10 pounds (4.5 kg) — sometimes more — in the first week of eating this way. This weight loss includes both body fat and water weight.
- One study in healthy women with obesity reported that a very low carb diet was more effective than a low fat diet for short-term weight loss (4Trusted Source).
- Research suggests that a low carb diet can reduce appetite, which may lead you to eat fewer calories without thinking about it or feeling hungry (5).
- Put simply, reducing carbs can lead to quick, easy weight loss.

<u>summary</u>

Removing sugars and starches, or carbs, from your diet can reduce your appetite, lower your insulin levels, and make you lose weight without feeling hungry.

<u>**2. Eat protein, fat, and vegetables**</u>

- Each one of your meals should include a protein source, fat source, and low carb vegetables.
- As a general rule, try eating two to three meals per day. If you find yourself hungry in the afternoon, add a fourth meal.
- Constructing your meals in this way should bring your carb intake down to around 20–50 grams per day.
- To see how you can assemble your meals, check out this low carb meal plan and list of 101 healthy low carb recipes.

- Protein
- Eating plenty of protein is an essential part of this plan.
- Evidence suggests that eating lots of protein may boost calorie expenditure by 80–100 calories per day (6Trusted Source, 7Trusted Source, 8Trusted Source).
- High protein diets can also reduce cravings and obsessive thoughts about food by 60%, reduce the desire to snack late at night by half, and make you feel full. In one study, people on a higher protein diet ate 441 fewer calories per day (9Trusted Source, 10Trusted Source).
- When it comes to losing weight, protein is a crucial nutrient to think about.
- Healthy protein sources include:

Meat: beef, chicken, pork, and lamb
Fish and seafood: salmon, trout, and shrimp
Eggs: whole eggs with the yolk
Plant-based proteins: beans, legumes, and soy

<u>Low carb vegetables</u>

- Don't be afraid to load your plate with low carb vegetables. They are packed with nutrients and you can eat very large amounts without going over 20–50 net carbs per day.
- A diet based mostly on lean protein sources and vegetables contains all the fiber, vitamins, and minerals you need to be healthy.
- Many vegetables are low in carbs, including:
- broccoli
- cauliflower
- spinach
- tomatoes
- kale

- Brussels sprouts
- cabbage
- Swiss chard
- lettuce
- cucumber
- See a full list of low carb vegetables here.
- Healthy fats
- Don't be afraid of eating fats. Trying to do low carb and low fat at the same time can make sticking to the diet very difficult.
- Sources of healthy fats include:
- olive oil
- coconut oil
- avocado oil
- butter
- summary
- Assemble each meal out of a protein source, fat source, and low carb vegetables. This will generally put you in a carb range of 20–50 grams and significantly lower your hunger levels.
- **<u>3. Lift weights three times per week</u>**
- You don't need to exercise to lose weight on this plan, but it will have extra benefits.
- By lifting weights, you will burn lots of calories and prevent your metabolism from slowing down, which is a common side effect of losing weight (11, 12Trusted Source).
- Studies on low carb diets show that you can gain a bit of muscle while losing significant amounts of body fat (13).
- Try going to the gym three to four times a week to lift weights. If you're new to the gym, ask a trainer for some advice.

- If lifting weights is not an option for you, doing some cardio workouts like walking, jogging, running, cycling, or swimming will suffice. Both cardio and weightlifting can help with weight loss.

summary

Resistance training, such as weight lifting, may be the best option. If that's not possible, cardio workouts are also effective.

ADVERTISEMENT

<u>Start a custom weight loss program</u>

- Noom helps you adopt healthy habits so you can lose weight and keep it off. Your program is customized towards your goals and fitness needs. Just take a quick assessment and get started today.
- Try doing a 'carb refeed' once per week
- If you need to, you can take one day off per week where you eat more carbs. Many people choose to do this on Saturday.
- It's important to stick to healthy carb sources like oats, rice, quinoa, potatoes, sweet potatoes, and fruit. If you must have a cheat meal and eat something unhealthy, do it on this day.
- Limit this to one higher carb day per week. If you aren't reducing carbs enough, you might not experience weight loss.
- You might gain some water weight during your refeed day, and you will generally lose it again in the next 1–2 days.

summary

- Having one day each week where you eat more carbs is acceptable, although not necessary.
- What about calories and portion control?
- It's not necessary to count calories as long as you keep your carb intake very low and stick to protein, fat, and low carb vegetables.
- However, if you want to count them, you can use a free online calculator like this one.
- Enter your sex, weight, height, and activity levels. The calculator will tell you how many calories to eat per day to maintain your weight, lose weight, or lose weight fast.
- You can also download free, easy-to-use calorie counters from websites and app stores. Here is a list of 5 calorie counters to try.

summary

It's not necessary to count calories to lose weight on this plan. It's most important to strictly keep your carbs in the 20–50-gram range.

10 weight loss tips

<u>Here are 10 more tips to lose weight faster:</u>

- Eat a high protein breakfast. Eating a high protein breakfast could reduce cravings and calorie intake throughout the day (16Trusted Source, 17Trusted Source).
- Avoid sugary drinks and fruit juice. These are among the most fattening things you can put into your body (18Trusted Source, 19).
- Drink water before meals. One study showed that drinking water a half hour before meals increased weight loss by 44% over 3 months (20Trusted Source).

- Choose weight-loss-friendly foods. Some foods are better for weight loss than others. Here is a list of 20 healthy weight-loss-friendly foods.
- Eat soluble fiber. Studies show that soluble fibers may promote weight loss. Fiber supplements like glucomannan can also help (21Trusted Source, 22Trusted Source).
- Drink coffee or tea. Caffeine boosts your metabolism by 3–11% (23Trusted Source, 24Trusted Source, 25Trusted Source).
- Base your diet on whole foods. They are healthier, more filling, and much less likely to cause overeating than processed foods.
- Eat slowly. Eating quickly can lead to weight gain over time, while eating slowly makes you feel more full and boosts weight-reducing hormones (26, 27Trusted Source).
- Weigh yourself every day. Studies show that people who weigh themselves every day are much more likely to lose weight and keep it off for a long time (28Trusted Source, 29Trusted Source).
- Get good quality sleep. Sleep is important for many reasons, and poor sleep is one of the biggest risk factors for weight gain (30).

- Sticking to the three-step plan allows for quick weight loss, and using other tips will make the diet plan even more effective.
- How fast will you lose weight?
- You may lose 5–10 pounds (2.3–4.5 kg) of weight — sometimes more — in the first week of the diet plan, and then lose weight consistently after that.

- If you're new to dieting, weight loss may happen more quickly. The more weight you have to lose, the faster you will lose it.
- For the first few days, you might feel a bit strange. Your body is used to running off carbs, and it can take time for it to get used to burning fat instead.
- Some people experience the "keto flu," or "low carb flu." It's usually over within a few days.
- After the first few days, most people report feeling very good, with even more energy than before.
- Aside from weight loss, the low carb diet can improve your health in many ways:
- blood sugar levels tend to significantly decrease on low carb diets (31)
- triglycerides tend to go down (32Trusted Source)
- LDL (bad) cholesterol goes down (33Trusted Source, 34)
- HDL (good) cholesterol goes up (35Trusted Source)
- blood pressure improves significantly (36Trusted Source, 37)
- low carb diets can be as easy to follow as low fat diets
- summary
- Most people lose a significant amount of weight on a low carb diet, but the speed depends on the individual. Low carb diets also improve certain markers of health, such as blood sugar and cholesterol levels.

The bottom line

- By reducing carbs and lowering insulin levels, you'll likely experience reduced appetite and hunger. This removes the main reasons it's often difficult to maintain a weight loss plan.

- On this plan, you can likely eat healthy food until you're full and still lose a significant amount of fat. The initial drop in water weight can lead to a drop in the scales within a few days. Fat loss takes longer.
- Studies comparing low carb and low fat diets suggest that a low carb diet might even make you lose up to two to three times as much weight as a typical low fat, calorie-restricted diet (38, 39, 40Trusted Source).
- If you have type 2 diabetes, talk to your healthcare provider before making changes, as this plan can reduce your need for medication.
- If you want to try a low carb diet, check out these 7 healthy low carb meals that you can make in 10 minutes or less.

Read this article in Spanish.
ADVERTISEMENT
Start a custom weight loss program

Noom helps you adopt healthy habits so you can lose weight and keep it off. Your program is customized towards your goals and fitness needs. Just take a quick assessment and get started today.

Last medically reviewed on March 5, 2020
Written by Kris Gunnars, BSc on March 5, 2020 — Medically reviewed by Atli Arnarson BSc, PhD
related stories

26 Weight Loss Tips That Are Actually Evidence-Based
20 Common Reasons Why You're Not Losing Weight
How Many Carbs Should You Eat per Day to Lose Weight?
16 Ways to Motivate Yourself to Lose Weight
How Walking Can Help You Lose Weight and Belly Fat
How to Lose Weight Fast: 3 Simple Steps, Based on Science

10 Morning Habits That Help You Lose Weight

29 Healthy Snacks That Can Help You Lose Weight

How Intermittent Fasting Can Help You Lose Weight

The 14 Best Ways to Burn Fat Fast

Was this article helpful?

Yes

No

Read this next

26 Weight Loss Tips That Are Actually Evidence-Based

Medically reviewed by Kris Gunnars, BSc

Most weight loss methods are unproven and ineffective. Here is a list of 26 weight loss tips that are actually supported by real scientific studies.

READ MORE

20 Common Reasons Why You're Not Losing Weight

Medically reviewed by Kris Gunnars, BSc

This article lists 20 common reasons why you're not losing weight. Many people stop losing before they reach a weight they are happy with.

READ MORE

How Many Carbs Should You Eat per Day to Lose Weight?

Medically reviewed by Kris Gunnars, BSc

Reducing carbohydrates in the diet is a great way to lose weight and improve health. This page explains how many carbs you should aim for each day.

READ MORE

16 Ways to Motivate Yourself to Lose Weight

Medically reviewed by Caroline Pullen, MS, RD

Here are 16 effective ways you can motivate yourself to lose weight. People often lack the motivation to get started or continue on a weight loss diet.

READ MORE

How Walking Can Help You Lose Weight and Belly Fat

Medically reviewed by Helen West, RD (UK)

Walking is a great form of physical activity that's free, low risk and easy to do. Importantly, it can also help you lose weight and belly fat.

READ MORE

A 7-Step Plan to Lose 10 Pounds in Just One Week

Medically reviewed by Rudy Mawer, MSc, CISSN

Sometimes you may need to lose a lot of weight quickly. Here is a 7-step plan to lose 10 pounds in just a week, backed by science.

READ MORE

12 Popular Weight Loss Pills and Supplements Reviewed

Medically reviewed by Kris Gunnars, BSc

This is a detailed, evidence-based review of the 12 most popular weight loss pills and supplements on the market today.

READ MORE

Can Omega-3 Fish Oil Help You Lose Weight?

Medically reviewed by Alina Petre, MS, RD (NL)

The omega-3 fatty acids in fish oil have many potential health benefits, including weight loss. This article examines whether omega-3 fish oil can...

READ MORE

11 Foods to Avoid When Trying to Lose Weight

Medically reviewed by Hrefna Palsdottir, MS

Some foods are proven to help you lose weight, while others make you gain. Here are 11 foods to avoid when trying to lose weight.

READ MORE

- Why Eggs Are a Killer Weight Loss Food
- Medically reviewed by Adda Bjarnadottir, MS, RDN (Ice)

- Whole eggs are among the best foods for weight loss. They are high in nutrients and help make you feel full, among other benefits.

READ MORE

Get our wellness newsletter

Filter out the noise and nurture your inbox with health and wellness advice that's inclusive and rooted in medical expertise.A 7-Step Plan to Lose 10 Pounds in Just One Week

If you buy something through a link on this page, we may earn a small commission. How this works.

If you want to lose 10 pounds (4.5 kg) in one week, then you need to follow an effective plan.

I've tested this plan on clients who were looking to lose weight fast before an event like a vacation or photo shoot, and it works wonders.

In fact, some of my clients who use this look like they've been on a three- or four-week diet after just one week.

Although it's not a long-term fix, this can kick-start your weight loss journey and motivate you for more sustainable long-term changes.

This plan is not recommended if you have a history of eating disorders like anorexia.

It Is Possible to Lose 10 Pounds in a Week

While it's certainly possible to lose 10 lbs in one week, it won't be pure body fat.

Due to the calorie deficit needed to burn each pound of fat, it's simply not possible to safely burn 10 pounds of pure body fat in just one week.

However, this isn't to say you can't lose that much weight and still look leaner.

While a lot of the weight loss will certainly come from body fat, you will also drop pounds by losing excess water weight (1Trusted Source).

This is partly because this plan lowers your insulin levels and makes your body get rid of stored carbs, which bind water.

Although your body can only store about 300–500 grams of carbs in a form known as glycogen, stored glycogen does hold around three times that weight in water (1Trusted Source, 2Trusted Source).

Reduced insulin levels will also make your kidneys shed out excess sodium, leading to reduced water retention (3Trusted Source, 4Trusted Source).

Along with reduced body fat and water weight, you may also lose some weight due to less intestinal waste and undigested food and fiber in the digestive system.

<u>Here are the 7 steps you should follow in order to lose 10 pounds in a week.</u>

<u>1. Eat Fewer Carbs and More Lean Proteins</u>

- You can lose several pounds by following a low-carb diet for just a few days.
- In fact, lots of research has shown a low-carb diet is a very effective way to lose weight and improve health (5Trusted Source, 6Trusted Source, 7Trusted Source).
- A short-term decrease in carb intake can also reduce water weight and bloating.
- This is why people who go low-carb often see a difference on the scale as early as the next morning after starting the diet.
- Additionally, making sure you eat plenty of protein can help reduce your appetite even further while boosting your metabolism (8Trusted Source, 9Trusted Source).

- Try eliminating or drastically reducing all starchy carbs and sugars for the week. Replace these with low-carb vegetables, while also increasing your intake of eggs, lean meats and fish.
- Check out this article to learn more about how to set up a low-carb diet and which foods to include.

<u>Bottom Line:</u>
Reducing your carb intake can lead to a significant amount of weight loss, from both body fat and excess water weight. Eating more protein also helps.

<u>2. Eat Whole Foods and Avoid Most Processed Junk Foods</u>

- When you're trying to lose weight quickly then it can be helpful to eat a simple diet based on whole foods.
- These foods tend to be very filling, and make it easier to eat fewer calories without getting too hungry.
- During the week, you should make sure to eat mostly whole, single-ingredient foods. Avoid most foods that are highly processed.
- Eating mostly lean proteins and low-carb veggies can be incredibly satisfying even if you're not getting that many calories.

Bottom Line:
In order to help you achieve the 10 pound goal, then you should try to eat only whole foods during this week. Base most of your diet on lean protein and low-carb veggies.

<u>Healthline Challenges</u>
Want to feel full without going on a diet? Take our free 21 day challenge

Change your relationship with your food by focusing on a new aspect of mindful eating each day. Join our nutrition newsletter for 21 days of mindful eating!

Your privacy is important to us

<u>3. Reduce Your Calorie Intake by Following These Tips (See List)</u>

- Reducing your calorie intake may be the most important factor when it comes to weight loss.
- If you aren't eating fewer calories than you expend, then you will not lose fat (10Trusted Source).
- Here is a calculator that shows you how many calories you should eat to lose weight (opens in new tab).

Here are a few simple tips to reduce calorie intake:

- Count calories: Weigh and log the foods you eat. Use a calorie counting tool to keep track of the amount of calories and nutrients you are taking in.
- Eat only at meals: Reduce all snacks and don't eat anything after dinner.
- Cut your condiments: Eliminate calorie-dense condiments and sauces.
- Fill up on veggies: Fill your plate with vegetables and limit starchy carbs and added fats for the week.
- Choose lean proteins: Choose lower-fat proteins, such as chicken and fish.
- Don't drink your calories: Instead, opt for water, zero-calorie drinks, tea or coffee. Protein shakes are fine if you count them as a meal.

Bottom Line:

Reducing your calorie intake is a vital factor for weight loss.

You may need to do this aggressively in order to lose so much weight in just one week.

<u>4. Lift Weights and Try High-Intensity Interval Training</u>

- Exercise is one of the best ways to burn fat and improve your appearance.
- Resistance training, such as weight lifting, can lead to a similar amount of weight loss as regular aerobic training. It also helps you add or maintain muscle mass and strength (11Trusted Source, 12Trusted Source).
- Full-body resistance training workouts are also a great method to lower your body's carb stores and water weight, which can lead to a sharp decline in weight (13Trusted Source, 14Trusted Source).
- Lifting weights can also protect your metabolism and hormone levels, which often decline during dieting (15Trusted Source, 16Trusted Source).
- High-intensity interval training (HIIT) is another very effective training method.
- Research suggests that 5–10 minutes of HIIT can lead to similar or greater benefits for health and weight loss as five times that amount of regular exercise (17Trusted Source, 18Trusted Source, 19Trusted Source).
- Like weight lifting, it can quickly reduce muscle carb stores and also boost other important aspects of weight loss, such as your metabolism and fat-burning hormones (20Trusted Source, 21Trusted Source).
- You can perform HIIT three to four times a week after a workout or as part of your normal training regimen. It is very important to do this with 100% effort or intensity. Most sprints should not last more than 30 seconds.
- Here are a few protocols you can try. These can be done running in place or outside, or applied to a cardio

machine like a bike, rower or treadmill:

- Session 1: 10 x 20-second sprint with 40 seconds rest
- Session 2: 15 x 15-second sprint with 30 seconds rest
- Session 3: 7 x 30-second sprint with 60 seconds rest
- Session 4: 20 x 10-second sprint with 20 seconds rest

Bottom Line:

Lifting weights and doing high-intensity intervals are among the best ways to lose weight and deplete muscle glycogen stores. They can also boost your metabolism and provide other benefits.

<u>5. Be Active Outside of the Gym</u>

- In order to burn extra calories and lose more weight, you can also increase your daily activity.
- In fact, how active you are throughout the day when you aren't exercising also plays a very important role in weight loss and obesity (22Trusted Source, 23Trusted Source).
- For example, the difference between a desk job and a manual job can account for up to 1,000 calories per day. This is the same as 90 to 120 minutes of high-intensity exercise (24Trusted Source).
- Simple lifestyle changes such as walking or biking to work, taking the stairs, going for walks outside, standing more or even cleaning the house can help you burn a lot of calories.

Bottom Line:

Increasing your daily activity is a great way to burn extra calories and lose more weight.

<u>6. Intermittent Fasting Is Another Simple Way to Reduce Weight Quickly</u>

- Intermittent fasting is another effective and proven tool for dropping fat (25Trusted Source, 26Trusted Source).
- It forces you to reduce your calorie intake, since you are limiting your eating to a short window of time.
- There are many different protocols, such as a 16-hour fast with an 8-hour feeding window, or a 20-hour fast with a 4-hour feeding window.
- If you're combining fasting with exercise, it may be wise to do the fasting at a different time than your workout.

Bottom Line:
Intermittent fasting is an excellent method to reduce calorie intake and lose weight.

<u>7. Use These Tips to Reduce Water Retention</u>

- Several other methods can help you drop water weight and appear leaner and lighter. These include:
- Take dandelion extract: A supplement called dandelion extract can help reduce water retention (27Trusted Source).
- Drink coffee: Coffee is a healthy source of caffeine. Studies suggest that caffeine can help you burn more fat and lose excess water (28Trusted Source).
- Mind your intolerances: Eating things that you are intolerant to, such as gluten or lactose, can lead to excessive water retention and bloating. Avoid foods that you think you may be intolerant to.
- Here are 13 more ways to lose excess water weight.

Bottom Line:
Other ways to lose water weight include supplementing with dandelion extract, drinking coffee and avoiding foods you are intolerant to.

<u>Take Home Message</u>

- By optimizing your diet and training regimen you can lose a large amount of weight in just one week.
- Although this won't be pure fat loss, it may give you the kick-start and motivation you need to follow a more sustainable diet.
- You do not need to follow all of these steps, but the more you apply, the more weight you will lose.
- Keep in mind that people who go on "crash diets" often end up gaining all the weight back when they're done.
- When the week is over, you should switch to a more sustainable plan so that you can continue to lose weight and keep it off.

<u>11 Ways to Stop Cravings for Unhealthy Foods and Sugar</u>

- The 20 Most Weight-Loss-Friendly Foods on The Planet
- 13 Easy Ways to Lose Water Weight (Fast and Safely)
- How Many Calories Should You Eat per Day to Lose Weight?
- How to Lose Weight Fast: 3 Simple Steps, Based on Science
- How to Lose Weight Fast: 3 Simple Steps, Based on Science
- 10 Morning Habits That Help You Lose Weight
- 29 Healthy Snacks That Can Help You Lose Weight
- How Intermittent Fasting Can Help You Lose Weight
- The 14 Best Ways to Burn Fat Fast
- Was this article helpful?

READ MORE

How Many Calories Should You Eat per Day to Lose Weight?

Medically reviewed by Kris Gunnars, BSc

Here's a simple but accurate calorie calculator that shows exactly how many calories you should eat to lose A 7-Step Plan to Lose 10 Pounds in Just One Week

If you buy something through a link on this page, we may earn a small commission. How this works.

If you want to lose 10 pounds (4.5 kg) in one week, then you need to follow an effective plan.

I've tested this plan on clients who were looking to lose weight fast before an event like a vacation or photo shoot, and it works wonders.

In fact, some of my clients who use this look like they've been on a three- or four-week diet after just one week.

Although it's not a long-term fix, this can kick-start your weight loss journey and motivate you for more sustainable long-term changes.

This plan is not recommended if you have a history of eating disorders like anorexia.

It Is Possible to Lose 10 Pounds in a Week

While it's certainly possible to lose 10 lbs in one week, it won't be pure body fat.

Due to the calorie deficit needed to burn each pound of fat, it's simply not possible to safely burn 10 pounds of pure body fat in just one week.

However, this isn't to say you can't lose that much weight and still look leaner.

While a lot of the weight loss will certainly come from body fat, you will also drop pounds by losing excess water weight (1Trusted Source).

This is partly because this plan lowers your insulin levels and makes your body get rid of stored carbs, which bind water.

Although your body can only store about 300–500 grams of carbs in a form known as glycogen, stored glycogen does hold around three times that weight in water (1Trusted Source, 2Trusted Source).

Reduced insulin levels will also make your kidneys shed out excess sodium, leading to reduced water retention (3Trusted Source, 4Trusted Source).

Along with reduced body fat and water weight, you may also lose some weight due to less intestinal waste and undigested food and fiber in the digestive system.

READ MORETake Home Message

By optimizing your diet and training regimen you can lose a large amount of weight in just one week.

Although this won't be pure fat loss, it may give you the kick-start and motivation you need to follow a more sustainable diet.

www.ingramcontent.com/pod-product-compliance
Lightning Source LLC
Chambersburg PA
CBHW051240250726
48656CB00003B/1055